I0423423

One Meal a Day:
A Breakthrough Diet
with
Health, Energy & Focus
(Seven Simple Steps to a
Fast Bulletproof Diet)

BEN FRANK

The best-selling author of "Positive Thinking Power: How to live a stress free life with confidence, happiness, and Joy (Five Simple Steps to Positive Lifestyle)"

www.thelifesuccess.com (coming soon)

*If you are sick or under prescribed medicine, please consult your physician or doctor before starting this diet.

ISBN: **1532870124**
ISBN-13: **978-1532870125**

DEDICATION

This book is dedicated to all the people fighting to lose weight.

After hearing about my success in diet, my father (age 70, Ph.D.) told me that he, too, wants to lose like 20 pounds. He survived two cancers and has been maintaining a healthy lifestyle (no alcohol, drugs, cigarettes, and coffee), but he wasn't losing any weight. Obviously he, too, had a voracious appetite like me! So, I gave him a copy this book. The first comment he gave me was this, "Hey, Ben, I am surprised that it didn't cost him a thing!"

I am trying to sell a product or anything here. I lost more than 20 pounds and did it mainly for health reasons. I thought anybody who tries to lose weight should enjoy the benefit that I gained. All I did was to read one good book and follow its advice. I am just doing the same to you hoping you do the same. Read this book, follow it thoroughly and write a better book than this only for the benefit of others.

Giving this book to my father, I told him how much I loved him and that I wish him to live a long happy life in good health. But I also told him that I can't help him lose his weight unless he changes his diet.

No matter how much you love your family and friends, you can't change other people's diet. Luckily, my dad followed my advice, and he lost 20 pounds after several months. He never gained any weight back. He is healthier and stronger than ever and says he will continue on with this diet forever.

CONTENTS

*If you are sick or under prescribed medicine, please consult your physician or doctor before starting this diet.

ACKNOWLEDGMENTS

I would like to thank my family, friends, and the publisher for helping me finish this book.

INTRODUCTION

I want to thank you and congratulate you for purchasing this book, "One Meal a Day: A Breakthrough Diet with Health, Energy, and Focus (Seven Simple Steps to a Fast Bulletproof Diet)"

Consisting of seven chapters, this book contains proven steps and strategies to lose weight and live an energetic life. Read this book and learn how to diet innovatively, motivate yourself and others constantly, and live a healthier and happier life.

Thanks again for purchasing this book. I hope you enjoy it!

Ben Frank

April 21st, 2016

QUICK SEVEN STEP APPROACH

Most studies are done on intermittent fasting, but that is not the subject of our discussion here. I am talking about one meal a day. In the past, the only time I fasted was during religious fasting days, or when cleansing my body with a body cleansing kit at the local pharmacies. Nowadays, I only eat one meal a day. I eat smaller amounts than before, and I am still healthy. Each day, I only get better at eating less. I am not bolemic or anorexic, and I don't have an eating disorder.

I started my diet after thoroughly reviewing a Japanese writer's book titled, "Being Hungry Makes You Healthy: One Meal a Day and You'll Look 20 Years Younger!" by Dr. Nagumo Yoshinori (南雲吉則) (http://www.booksfromjapan.jp/authors/item/1147-yoshinori-nagumo), a Japanese medical doctor, whose bestseller hit all over Asia. His principles can be summarized by these basic seven rules.

*Disclaimer: This book follows the basic principles, but Dr. Nagumo Yoshinori was not involved in the production of, and does not endorse this book product.

1. Eat whole foods
2. Enjoy the food as much as you can by eating it slowly
3. Avoid caffeinated drinks or energy drinks
4. Chew gums
5. Learn to enjoy fasting
6. Do not exercise excessively
7. Learn to sleep on an empty stomach.

1. Eat whole foods such as milk, soymilk, eggs, and whole fish. Westerners (Americans and Europeans) have a poor habit of eating meat because most of us only eat the flesh. We do not eat the skin, bones, or the heads. We only eat the tasty parts, which only get us fat by gaining excess partial nutrition namely, protein, sugar, and fat. Of course, the argument that primates like us have to eat the whole fish from eyeballs and intestines to the fish tail may sound ridiculous to us, but in many parts of Asia, they do so. Therefore, I suggest we eat as many different parts of fish or meat as possible. For example, eat the dark and white meat. Eat Asian style (Korean/Japanese) lightly fried, dried whole anchovies, shrimps or eat sardines and various kinds of fish like Europeans. Try different kinds of meat and fish rather than eating just chicken, pork, or beef.

2. Enjoy food as slowly as possible. One thing that you have to adapt eventually is the slow eating habit, which is excellent in many ways. First, we get to fully chew and digest what we eat, not to mention that we fully

savor the flavors. We also don't need to hurry as we are going to eat only one meal a day. Therefore, we can sit down, relax and enjoy. I mean you have to enjoy that one meal you get to eat in a day. You will wait and anticipate, meaning your body will be better prepared for a delightful meal and its full digestion.

3.   Avoid caffeinated drinks or energy drinks. Caffeine is a chemical produced by plants as a defense mechanism, so that herbivores may feel dizzy when they eat too much grass. Do other herbivore predators need caffeine? Then, why do we need caffeine? What about energy drinks? Later, I will explain, but energy boosts mean energy pit. Do not expect to get high without facing the valley. In order for us to maintain good body health and mentality, we need to avoid all kinds of stimulants. Personally, it was harder for me to quit coffee than tea. Knowing this, I moved from coffee to tea. Substance abuse or addition is never a good thing as your body depends on it. Once you depend on a substance, you lose control. Diet is all about control. So, do not lose control.

4.   Chew gums. I once met an old couple college professor from Princeton University at airport. We talked about the use of gums. Well, one thing I learned from them was the act of chewing helps blood circulation in the brain. This couple was studying about the brain and had knowledge

about it. Now, the reason why I believe chewing a gum is necessary is because it is a low calorie substitute for candies and it suppresses your hunger. I enjoy cinnamon or mint gums. I chew two to four sticks of gum per day and it has been very helpful. I stop when my jaws hurt. Remember that you have a long wait for your next meal (the next day), so you better get used to chewing a gum.

5.   Learn to enjoy fasting. As many of you already know, the part that does all the logic and calculations of the portion you have to eat is your brain. It tells you, "Oh, you can eat this, you have done it before." What this means is, dieting is going to be hard. You have to be mentally armed and sharp to do it right. One meal a day means you have to restrict your diet. Many people who practice one meal a day say that you can eat all what you want in one meal. This always works, because I eat like crazy. My wife, my children, my co-workers and the managers of my favorite restaurants know I eat much in one meal. The rest of the time, (the time you do not eat) will make your stomach smaller. So, eventually the amount that you eat (your appetite) and your measure of what you can eat will be reduced. In other words, you will know that your body can only eat less each month. You will soon realize that you can eat small amount of food and learn to enjoy it.

6.   Do not exercise excessively. Anything excessive is never good. Now your main concern in life is health. It is not work productivity, even though your productivity will eventually improve, as you get healthier. Your relationship, love, money, and all the rest will only improve when your body feels better. Excessive exercise can result in muscle pain, exhaustion, and injuries. It also consumes a minimum of two to three hours per day from start to end (including shower and changing clothes), not to mention the nap you might have to take afterwards. Another reason I am against this is that it makes you even hungrier. Exercise expedites your digestion, meaning you get hungry fast. If you are taking one meal a day, you do not have to feel like your hunger is going to last forever. Exercising is not bad as long as it is done moderately, but it is not necessary.

7.   Learn to sleep on an empty stomach. The best part about one meal a day program is that you can sleep like a baby. You feel like you are rejuvenated every morning. No One bad habit we all learn living in this human world is sleeping on full stomach. This bad habit begins when we are born. Mommies feed the babies to sleep. When we grow up, we eat, drink, and party to sleep. How do we feel the next day? Lousy, right? Waking up with a crystal clear mind without any aches, migraines, muscle pains, stomach problems, and circulation problems is important. However, you do not need coffee in the morning to wake yourself up. That's not how

we used to wake before we all started to drink coffee, tea, or any other drinks. Start this diet and you will wake up wake up earlier than normal. Start making your first batch of barley tea (Barley tea is not really a normal tea, as it contains no caffeine. It is a barley drink) or warm soymilk or milk. You can easily get a barley tea bag at an Asian market or order them from the Internet. I got mine from a local Korean market. When I first started this diet, I used to sleep around ten and usually got up around four or five. These days, I get up around five or six. Nowadays, I only sleep six hours a day and I feel great. I feel energized as ever, the way it should be.

CHAPTER 1
LOSE 4-10 POUNDS IMMEDIATELY (PHASE 1)

Want a fast diet? Here it is. Lose 4-10 pounds immediately.

1.   One of the fastest ways to lose weight is through fasting. I am not telling you to not eat anything for a week, but if you could, skip dinner or breakfast. If you could do it for a week or two, you will lose 4-10 pounds in your first month. It happened so fast and I lost so much weight! However, I had nothing to worry because I was eating enough food and I felt like it too. I was hungry, but I could feel that my stomach was getting smaller and flatter. My waistline was getting smaller, my circulation was better with cholesterol level slightly going down, and my liver (GOP and GTP) levels improved fast too.

2.   Beginner's luck, if you read Paulo Coelho's novel, "The Alchemist" you definitely know what I mean. It is a God given gift for starters taking

on a personal legend or a life long journey to find treasure. In our case, it would be success in diet. It is your first jackpot in a lottery or your first win in a gamble. I dare say you should enjoy it while it lasts.

3.   Why? Because it soon scares you. True, winning with lots of possibilities involved scares people later on. Trust me; diet has more to do with your mind than anything else does. Unless you are big, fat, or obese due to medical reasons, then it is mainly because of your mental and social matters. If you win once and continue to win without much effort, you will soon think that it is boring. Diet is never like that. We know how hard it is. Especially when you age, it only gets harder to lose weight. It is just like life, it only gets tougher to fight. You might as well enjoy it while you are victorious.

4.   Actually, the first time I lost weight through fasting, happened when I was in high school. It was my first diet and I had to fast for one week. I did not eat for three days and I lost weight so fast that it scared me. If you are young, the effect of fasting is greater because your metabolism is higher. However, after three days I got scared. I had already lost 10 pounds by then, and I lost my appetite too. For the first two days, I did not eat anything. Only on the third day did I drink some water. I thought I might die, so I slowly started eating again with porridge. My stomach hurt a bit,

but I soon recovered. My weight shot up again as soon as I started eating again.

5.   So, what is my point? Don't be afraid of the bodily changes. If you had a diet before, you won't be scared. If this is your first time, you might be scared after losing so much weight within days, weeks, or even months. The effect is great at first. Enjoy it while it lasts. Think positively, especially when your body conditions improve. Your body will cherish it, and so will you. It is a blessing and it is great!

6.   If this is your first time going on a diet, it may be hard for you to skip meals or to eat small portions. I still find it extremely hard to eat smaller amounts per meal when there is a plenty of food to eat. My stomach grumbles as a signal that I need more food. However, you should learn to recognize when your body starts to lose weight. Every morning you wake up feeling your stomach getting flatter and hungry that is an indication you are losing weight. Every morning you wake up feeling awful and seem to have a circulation problem that is an alarm, you are gaining weight.

7.   One very important key to success in a diet is sustainability. Is your diet sustainable and for how long? I could not handle my total fasting in high school for more than three days. I knew I could really lose some

weight, but I gave up because I knew I couldn't fast forever.

8.   Another important key to success in a diet is your adaptability. What would you do when you wake up at 1 or 3am in the morning because you are hungry? This will actually happen to most of us when we start skipping dinner. How would you adjust your schedule to be more productive when you skip meals? What would you do for the free hours you get?

9.   The moment people realize something bad is going to happen, they tend to give up. Well, that's bad. My trick is not to use any trick. Just be truthful to yourself. Work on a way that truly works. Believe in it and live your life the way you designed it. It really works!

10.   To sum up, skip your breakfast or dinner. Skipping dinner (stop eating before six pm) works great. It is a fast, healthy way of losing weight. Skipping breakfast doesn't work so well, but works as a great accelerator when you do it with skipping dinner. Drink a lot of water to fill up your hunger. Do this for one month. I weighed 202 pounds when I started. Then, I lost 15pounds in one month (4 weeks)! Good luck!

     Email me about your success story after your first month weight loss. What is your name? Where are you from? How many pounds (or kg) did you lose in your first month? Are you happy? What's your next goal? I can be reached at thelifesuccess1@gmail.com.

CHAPTER 2
FIGHT YOUR HUNGER (PHASE 2)

Here is my secret to diet success. You are about to engage in a revolutionary lifestyle.

1. Let me tell you what I do. I am a researcher/instructor and have a Ph.D. but not a medical degree. Therefore, I am an average person when it comes to diet. I am in my early forties. My wife is a nutritionist (with a Ph.D.) but she and I live on different diets. She eats three very small meals a day with snacks and coffee. I on contrary eat one meal a day.

2. This kind of difference is actually very common among practitioners. Dr. Nagumo Yoshinori's wife or his other family members don't practice what he does and the family just works great. I too, have children and I don't tell them to go on my diet as they are too young. I think one should be at least 20 years old or older to practice dieting. This new program will be your friend forever.

3.   I take multi-vitamins and vitamin C (1000mg) every day. I do not take any medication. I weigh myself more than three times a day (twice in the morning and once at night) with a gym quality weight scale ($300 or more) and keep records of my body fat and muscles.

4.   In the morning, I drink one or two warm cups of thick almond milk, soymilk or milk. I sometimes add various freshly ground toasted crops (sesame seeds, black beans, soybeans, perilla seeds, sticky rice, rice, brown rice, oats or any other excellent grain mixes), but this is not necessary. I eat one or two bars of chocolate (34g each). It can be dark chocolate or milk chocolate, but I try to stick to one particular brand that is readily available. That way I can easily count the calories and maintain my diet anywhere I travel.

5.   In terms of the calories for my breakfast, two bars of chocolate and two cups of warm milk is equal to one light meal when we count the calories. However, it is better than bacons, sausages, ham and eggs or a full meal (breakfast buffet at a hotel) because it does not make you feel tired. Liquid diet works because liquids do not drain your energy unlike solid foods. This way, you can use the unused energy in digesting excessive energy that ultimately gets stored in your body as fat.

6. Throughout the day, to fight my hunger, I drink a lot of various warm non-caffeinated crop-based tea, such as barley, corn, and others, usually as much as half a gallon (1-2 liters). Warm drinks keep your body temperature warm, helping you to burn more calories. Crop based tea keep you healthy and keeps your stomach full more than water. You can boil it with less water and can drink it thick, but it still has little or no calories. I may drink black tea, green tea from time to time, but I do not drink coffee at all.

7. I eat lunch at noon and can eat anything any amount I want. In the past, I used to pile up food and eat like crazy. My lunch varies according to what my body wants. I can eat seafood, beef or vegetables. Usually, I eat many different kinds of food. I try not to fill my full meal with one extreme thing or two. I try to avoid eating donuts, sweets, chocolates, fatty food, or greasy food to extremes. I can do this but consciously.

8. After lunch, I take a 30 min. to one-hour nap. I usually do not eat dinner but try to accommodate friends and myself for certain occasions. If that is the case, I skip lunch and eat dinner instead. These days are somewhat hard so I drink juice or tea to keep myself less hungry. This usually happens once a week or once a month. You should be able to change your mealtime occasionally to make your diet sustainable.

9.   Usually I go to bed early around 10 or 11pm on an empty stomach. My latest bedtime is midnight. I crash on an empty stomach. When I am hungry and cannot get to sleep because of that, I drink barley tea or drink water and I sleep like a baby. I wake up in the morning feeling totally rejuvenated. I eat only one full meal a day.

10.   Most articles that I have read on longevity all seem to say that people who live close to 100 or more either eat one meal a day, two meals a day or three light meals a day. None of them eats to extremes. They also keep their meal times accurately. These people are also good at sustaining a healthy diet for a long time and so should we.

11.   You cannot use too many variations on what you can eat. For example, you cannot simply add or subtract what you eat for at least first two or three months. If you eat many different kinds of food, you only confuse your body. This is very important. If you change what you eat, you are strain. Therefore, you have to go steady until your body gets used to it. Trust me it takes time weeks or months to tame your body to follow your lead. Do not let it panic by frequently changing your diet. Go steady at first and slowly experiment and change what you eat.

12.   To sum it up, in order to make it a life long diet, you have to do something that is sustainable. I do liquid diet in the morning and eat one full meal a day. I drink one to two cups of warm soymilk or milk with powdered crops, and eat a chocolate bar or two. When I have dinner dates, I drink juices or tea in the afternoon and eat dinner. I go to bed early around 10pm. First, focus on going on a steady diet.

CHAPTER 3: CHEATING IS OKAY

Cheating is okay as long as you realize what it does. Cheat only when you have to. And when you cheat, use it to your advantage.

Obviously, you do not have to cheat, if you are such a strong willed person. I do not have a strong will. I am an average person when it comes to food. Actually, I love food and that is why I could not be successful in my diet for a long time. However, I have learned several ways to use cheating to my advantage.

1.   When do I cheat? I used to cheat a lot in the first three months. Now, I just do not cheat at all, because I do not have any reason to. Of course, when I do cheat, I count the calories. In the morning, when I am hungry, I drink two cups of warm milk instead of one. If I cannot wait until lunch, I eat two chocolate bars (of the same brand) instead of one. I drink crop-based tea more often.

2. I have a big Japanese tea thermos (1gallon/2.2 liters) in my office and freshly brew crop based tea at least once a day. I always surround myself with various kinds of tea to keep myself less hungry. Sometimes, when I am on a lunch date and do not eat enough, I have to eat more after the dinner to fill my empty stomach. If you do not fill up your stomach, snacking during the day is advisable.

3. However, there is one true DONT. That is snacking at night. This is something I rarely ever did. Eating late or eating in the middle of the night is something you should totally avoid. Whether you saw this on TV or what, it is very unhealthy and it ruins your diet. This may force you to start all over again. This is also something that I have never done in my entire practice. The key to success is not to eat after 6pm.

4. When I cheated, I gave myself a limit. That was once or twice a week, never thrice. Sometimes over the weekend when families gather, I usually try to have family gatherings for lunch rather than dinner, because then, I would not have to starve until dinnertime. Nowadays, I do not like eating dinner, but family circumstances force you to spend time with them, right? The time is so precious that you have to value the opportunity and really enjoy it.

5.   So, when unexpected family gatherings occurred, I ended up eating dinner. Therefore, I would eat lunch and dinner. Sometimes when I got up very hungry, I would eat for me to sleep. I did breakfast and lunch. I ate a lot back then. However, I never gorged myself three full meals. Usually, one meal (either lunch or dinner) was full, and the other was more of a snack. I just ate something very light to fill my stomach. I did that for three months.

6.   After the fourth month, I could really stick to my one meal diet. I knew and my body knew what would happen if I cheated. I would have a "very bad" sleep as opposed to "great" sleep. I could really compare the two. Slowly, I became distant from "very bad" sleep. It was great.

7.   Another advantage that I saw from these cheatings was at my medical checkups. After several months, my levels were not improving at all. When I took the blood test at the hospital, all my other levels (liver, blood pressure, and the rest) were down, but my weight and my cholesterol levels were not decreasing at all. Only then did I realize that I had to do something about it.

8.   As you continue to sleep with an empty stomach at night, you gradually decrease your stomach size and you can only eat less as days go

by. Therefore, instead of drinking two cups of warm milk, I could eat only one. Then, instead of cheating, I could just eat the chocolate when I was extremely hungry in the afternoon.

9.   Now, the greatest advantage of you taking things slowly is that your expectations are limited. Unlike the first month when you enjoyed a great thrill in losing a lot of weight, the change is definitely slower, but it happens steadily. It is a good feeling and a safe one. Because, when you continue to lose weight at such an increased speed, you will begin to worry about your health, and you will start to eat again. You will regain your weight back.

10.   From your second or third month, expect to lose only four pounds a month. That is only a pound a week. In addition, you might experience weight fluctuations. This happens as you drink a lot of water. Water helps you with your circulation and cleanses your system. The less you eat, the cleaner your system gets. Do not be disappointed.

11.   To sum it up, cheating is okay as long as you know what you are doing. Cheat only to get by, and never to overdo anything. Only snack when you are hungry during the day, and never late at night. Fully enjoy your one full meal during the day. Eat only to fill the hunger. Try to get by your day until you go to sleep. Once you go to sleep, it is another win. This

is how you win. You take small victories until you get accustomed to them.

Later, you can add on to your previous victories.

CHAPTER 4: TRULY UNDERSTAND YOYO

Weigh yourself at least three times a day and understand what yoyo is all about.

There are three phases to this diet. Once you get used to one meal a day practice (phase 3), you should gradually slow down on your habit of overeating. Overeating is never good. Eat lunch to your satisfaction and fill your stomach. Then, when you are hungry, snack in the late afternoon (if you do not want to, you do not have to). This is wiser and healthier. Eating two or three small meals a day is fine as long as you don't overeat. Many people who live up to more than 100 practice this.

1.   Why is it important to weigh at least three times a day? To understand the weight differences, the causes of weight losses or gains, and take advantage or the yo-yo. I usually start my day early like around five or six in the morning. That is normal for a primitive man like me.

2.   The first thing I do is to weigh myself on the scale. I almost go nude to get an accurate measurement. Then, I drink a cup of barley tea or a glass of water and get to work in my computer, waiting for my body's bathroom signal.

3.   After doing my number one or two in bathroom, I weigh myself on the scale one more time. I get the difference. The difference is huge! Usually, I lose a quarter of a pound after number 1 or one or two pounds after number 2. Now, this is your true weight with nothing in your stomach. Take a photo of your weight as a record.

4.   Even though this is optional, I sometimes weigh myself after lunch just to see how much I gained for lunch. Then, after returning home from work in the evening, I weigh myself for the third time. This of course, I do after I go to the bathroom. Now, how much do you weigh? You would probably weigh more. It is okay. This is a yo-yo and it is a cycle.

5.   You eat and your weight increases. If you consume more than you eat, your weight decreases. Your body doesn't tell a lie. Make it honest. That way, you can experiment with your food and learn more about the causes of weight loss and gain. If you ate too much of something, felt great, and didn't gain weight, that's fine. However, if you ate very little and still gained

a lot, that's not good. As you have guessed, the oily, sweet, or salty food makes you fat.

6.   Also, spare your time to get advice from a health professional. When your body is honest, your health professionals' (nutritionist, doctor) advice works best. As they see positive changes in your body, they will try to help you more. Be honest to yourself and to your health professionals.

7.   To sum it up, you should weigh yourself on the scale at least three to four times a day. That way you will notice body weight fluctuations depending on the time of day, and before and after meals. This way, you can train your mind and body to communicate honestly.

CHAPTER 5: TRAIN YOUR BODY TO TELL THE TRUTH

Your body can take almost anything when you are young and healthy. What you have is a buffer.

1.   Of course, you can train your body to lie. Our body system is so smart that it lies and you won't even know it. You hear skinny people brag about gorging high calorie drinks or food the other daily and claim they did not gain any weight. They think it is a heroic tale, but I call it an unhealthy tale.

2.   If you actually understand how much your body does to support your system, your poor eating and sleeping habits, you will be amazed at its resilience and recovering capacity. However, all these systems of yours eventually runs down over time and you will soon be left with an old house with leaking roof, broken windows, and a rickety door. This may sound sad, but it is the ultimate truth. We all live to run our very systems down. Some do it faster while others do it slower.

3.   I have a sad tale of a 74 years old diabetic patient, who has been on a very strict diet for the past thirty years since his first diagnosis. Every time I dine with him, I think he is an ascetic, but he still does not call himself a great ascetic. He says he still cheats sometimes. One day he shared his story with me of how and what he ate in his youth and it went like this.

4.   Everyday, he had five cans of soda, ate hamburgers, ice cream and cakes for desserts, meat, meat soup, and barbecues and alcohol at night. However, he still woke up and went to work the next day. It was hard for him, but he did it for twenty years.

5.   At first, he did not gain any weight, so he continued the habit for five to ten years. His buffer began to wear out early. When you are young and healthy, you have a good buffer zone that can support your crazy lifestyle. You don't seem to gain any weight after a night of heavy booze, food, and partying.

6.   If you do that occasionally, then your buffer recovers slowly. The recovery can be days, weeks or months. Remember that this "buffer" is a very abstract term and everyone's specific body conditions are different and unique. Just like how some people are born strong and when some are born

weak.

7.　If you are born healthy, your organ only fails when you abuse it. Once you use up all your buffers, then, you become vulnerable. While the buffer is active, your body can tell a lie. Once you pass that physical buffer (or your limit), you become chronic. You feel fatigue every morning, your body aches, and you have problems in your stomach, heart, skin, liver, and circulation.

8.　On top of all this, you act mean to others. You affect the lives of those close to you negatively. You become unhealthy and mean person or a good-natured obese person.

9.　Going back to our story, this old man's buffer was worn out. The doctor told him that his cholesterol level, GOP, and GTP were off the charts. His pancreas was not functioning properly. It was broken down for good and could never be fixed. Ever since then, he has been on a strict diet with medication. When do you realize the value of life or happiness? Only when you start to lose it.

10.　A new definition of health: You feel great everyday you wake up, you have no problems, you are free of pains, and chronic illnesses. Your medical report says you are healthy and normal. You sleep like a baby at night, and you have a very thick buffer for life's struggles and obstacles, which may arise at any time. Your life is without major worries of finance, job, relationships, and personal life. You are energetic, and you are nice to yourself and to others. You are willing to take risks and do not abuse your body in any way. You feel like you have tomorrow.

11.   The smaller you take, the more you get to enjoy life and the little things. Lengthen the fun and enjoyment by taking smaller bites out of food and life. When I first started this diet, I ate like crazy. I had a set goal, I woke up, and I stuffed my mouth with chocolate and soymilk. Then, I would worry until lunch, only to stuff myself with an enormous amount of food. Now, I no longer do that. I only eat moderately though I only eat once a day. It is perfectly fine for me. One meal a day is enough to run you through the whole day and night, not to mention it can help you rest.

12.   During your first week, you will lose weight rapidly. However, do not panic. During my first week, I lost 10 pounds and I was scared. I thought something bad was going to happen but only good things happened. My weight continuously decreased when my stamina (buffer) started to increase. I could work longer hours and sleep less. I could focus better. However, there was one drawback. I felt like I did not have enough energy.

13.   The truth of the matter is that you get energy boost when you overeat. It gets you high and you get a spike on your chart. However, hitting high means you will soon hit the deeper valley, which usually ends up in a crash. Sugar crash, exhaustion, poor circulation, and liver failure are only few of those symptoms that I can easily name. In other words, hitting high is never good. It does not help.

14.   Energy boosts and stimulants are not good. Just learn to take things slowly and steadily, moderation is the variety of life. When you overeat, your liver and stomach over function, taking away most of the blood and energy from other organs, making you feel lousier.

15.   If you are constantly binging, eating, and drinking, when does your body ever rest? You simply do not. You have to put your body to rest by not eating. By reducing the number of meals per day, you can also focus more on work and get more things done. Yes, there may be less extemporaneous fun, but more stability and strength and buffers. The more the buffer, the healthier you are.

16.   To sum up, you need to eat moderately and take things slowly. Overeating is never good. When it comes to eating habits, you think you are

changing one simple habit, but you are changing your whole life. Every time you treat your body right, you add another layer of buffer (stamina) to your system, ultimately lengthening your life expectancy.

6. THE THREE PHASES (PHASE 3)

Phase 3 is when you have no hunger strikes. Now, your stomach does not crave for food like it used to months ago. You may feel hunger when you do not eat your lunch on time, but you can handle the delay.

First, let me recap the phases a bit.
Phase 1: 1st month~
Phase 2: 2nd~4rd months
Phase 3: 5th Month~

Phase 1 should be your first month. You lose weight like fast and greatly. You can cheat and it is okay. It is a drastic change in life style anyway. Your body goes through fast changes. You wake up very early in the morning like 1 or 2AM in the morning. You do not know what to do. That is when you start your day. You may sometimes (like once or twice a week) eat breakfast because you woke up early out of hunger. It is the start of a new caveman style life.

Your health figures improve greatly. Especially, the liver levels will go down as your food intake goes down drastically. Your circulation problems will diminish. You may drink 100-200ml size (kid's size juice) or have light snacks like potato chips or half a sandwich to fight your hunger.

------------------If you stop here, you are losing to yoyo. Your health will go back to where it was. Actually, it will turn worse. That is what a yoyo does-- ----------------------

Phase 2 is the adaptation period where you still need to cheat from time to time. You still worry and have some doubts about the system. However, your cholesterol level should go down until it turns normal (less than 200mg/dl). You still lose weight, but not very much.

Your body is now very sensitive to the food that you eat. Therefore, it is a great time to experiment what kind of food gets you fat and what does not. For me it was the Chinese food (no offense) because I was eating too much sauce unlike the Chinese. Chinese people eat with chopsticks and avoid eating all the oily sauce. They just dip it lightly. You need to find your poor eating habits and fix them.

----------------------If you stop here, that is because you realize you cannot hold on to your old habits or hang out with your friends and families. However, you should never give in. Moreover, you can still hang out with them. You can actually do more for them--------------------

Phase 3 is the stabilization period where you no longer fight hunger. If you are still overweight, you will continue to lose weight (1-2 pounds per month) and your BMI (Body Mass Index) figure will continue to improve (less than 25%) until you say stop. You just know that it is not wise to cheat, so you do not cheat at all. You no longer need to drink tea, juice, or water. This is the time you start really understanding your body. Your body is under control. Food is no longer your priority in life. You are not interested in food and do not think about food as much. You only think about food once a day.

You are interested in yourself, your work and the people around you. You can truly focus on your life. You may be slightly overweight, but you are not worried about it. Because you know, you can handle it. You are also not worried about maintaining your healthy lifestyle. You continue it and take out more of the unnecessary parts such as chocolate or others. You try to improve your food intake by eating quality and nutritious food. You avoid oily food or any other unhealthy food, because your body knows it, and you understand it. You cannot really explain it why, but it just works that way.

Your stomach is smaller and weaker (meaning eating normal amounts) so you cannot handle the appetite you used to have months ago. You try, but you just cannot. You wake up fresh and you are ready for another great day.

You feel less under the weather, meaning your aches lessen or even disappear. You are no longer under the influence of the weather. Whether it is rainy, hot, or cold, you are still great, healthy, and happy you.

CHAPTER 7: THE SEVEN PRINCIPLES AND DIETING FOR LIFE

Now that you have trained your body to tell the truth, listen to your body. Eat what you feel like eating. Your body will tell you what to eat. Talk to your doctor. Go to a clinic and check your health on regular basis.

In the old days, diet meant, how you ate. Today, it just means, "to lose

weight." This is the wrong notion and everyone knows that.

We need to give this word its proper meaning back. You can do this by

saying the following to yourself.

"To diet means to eat and live well for the rest of my life."

People try to lose their weight overnight when it takes months and years for

them to gain weight. Shouldn't the reverse happen slowly? I think so and

phase three is all about this.

One answer that I found through this program was that diet is a series of life long habits. It is a lifestyle and you need to choose the right way to eat and live for the rest of your life.

I started this book with Dr. Nagumo Yoshinori's 7 principles.

1.   Eat whole foods
2.   Enjoy the food as much as you can by eating it slowly
3.   Avoid caffeinated drinks or energy drinks
4.   Chew gums
5.   Learn to enjoy fasting
6.   Do not exercise excessively
7.   Learn to sleep on an empty stomach.

At first, practicing these seven principles eating one meal a day seemed extremely hard. But now, this is what I do everyday. I no longer drink soda, coffee, or tea. My body knows they are not good for me. I don't overeat, I don't exercise to lose weight (just tone up my muscles.), and I sleep for at least four, six or eight hours.

All my levels (liver, cholesterol, blood pressure, sugar) are normal. I have no circulation problems, aches, or muscle pains. Even though I eat chocolate and chew gums, my teeth are fine. I have no problem going to family dinners or formal dinners. My friends, family and I still get along well even though I only eat lunch with them. I eat when I have to, but I don't when I don't need to.

I know how to fight hunger and I do it well. This alone takes away a lot of the stress that I used to have. I no longer think about food much or spend much time on food shopping. Now I have more time to spend on work, family, and on self-development. What are the chances of my life getting better? Very high.

This is why it is a breakthrough diet with health, energy, and focus. And it is a fast bulletproof diet.

Today, I am healthy, young, and happy and so should you.

One Meal a Day: A Breakthrough Diet with Health, Energy & Focus (Seven Simple Steps to a Fast Bulletproof Diet)

CONCLUSION

Thank you again for purchasing this book!

I hope this book gave you some ideas about losing your weight and regaining your health.

The next is to apply the principles into your daily life. Follow the simple steps given to you and that way you can lose weight fast and stay in good health.

Start inspiring and motivating people. Share this information with people who are close to you. Learn the value of one meal a day and influence other people to do the same. Remember this new diet is contagious. Always smile and let others see the positive things in this book.

Finally, if you enjoyed this book, please take the time to share your thoughts and post a review on Amazon. It'd be greatly appreciated!

Thank you and good luck!

BONUS 1: Positive Thinking Power: How to live a stress free life with confidence, happiness, and Joy (Five Simple Steps to Positive Lifestyle)

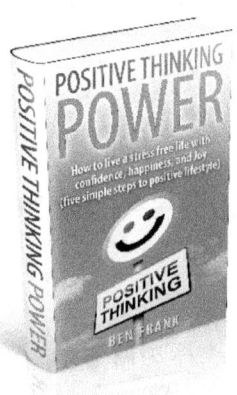

CHAPTER 5

POSITIVE DISCIPLINE: PRAISE YOURSELF AND OTHERS FOR THE ACCOMPLISHMENT OF A SPECIFIC TASK

"Praise yourself and others for the accomplishment of a specific task."

In this chapter, I have talked about positive discipline, which is how to discipline yourself and others. By focusing more on the positive sides and less on minor errors, we can move faster and with more energy towards our goals.

A professor of social psychology, Carol Dweck, at Stanford University conducted an experiment on fifth graders in an elementary school in New York. The children were first given an easy test. Since the questions were easy, all of the children did well, regardless of their usual grades. After their first test, two groups of children received similar scores, but the teacher praised the two groups differently.

Group A children were told, "You are so smart." In other words, the children were praised for their inborn ability or general intelligence. Group B children were told, "You worked really hard." Here, the children were praised for their effort.

Then there was the second test. This time, the students were given a choice to choose either the difficult test or the easy test. Surprisingly, most of the students who were praised for their general intelligence (Group A) chose the easy test. However, 90% of the children who were praised for their efforts (Group B) chose the difficult test.

The third test contained only difficult questions. Here, something more surprising happened. Those who were praised for their efforts (Group B) did their best and solved some of the difficult questions, whereas those who were praised for their intelligence (Group A) felt sad and disappointed by themselves after seeing the difficult questions.

The fourth test was the achievement test that measured how much these students improved from their first test. On this test, those who were praised for their efforts (Group B) improved their scores on average by 30% from their first test. However, those who were praised for their intelligence (Group A) on average scored 20% lower than their first test.

What does this experiment tell you? When you praise yourself, you need to recognize what you did right and how you worked for it. When you praise others, you should point out what they did right and how their efforts contributed to their success, not for some ability they might have been born with, such as general intelligence. This way you not only instill confidence and a sense of achievement, but you also leave some room for improvement. Then, you and others will want to think more creatively and actually try to do better on your next task.

Everyone fails. However, when you fail, do not beat yourself up or take out your anger on others. Think of creative measures for fast recovery. Do not focus on the negatives. Lead yourself and others to the next closest success with confidence and a positive attitude. Do not point out the negatives in others. As you spend more time helping others do well, people will in turn give more attention to you. After all, positive discipline is a habit.

1.   Only praise people for their achievements of specific tasks. Do not overpraise them or praise them for their intelligence or other talent. Praising people's inborn abilities often cripples them. Also, do not jump to conclusions and judge other people's intelligence or diligence in any manner.

2.   By profession, I am a teacher, but I am always trying to learn new things as a student. So, let me tell you a story. I once attended a motorcycle class because I really wanted to ride one well. I was an okay motorcyclist, but I wanted to feel safer out on the streets. It was a very tough two-day workshop. At the workshop, my instructor did not point out what I did wrong. He asked, "How did you make this turn?" Again, he only focused on praising what I did right and well. Thanks to him, I only focused on getting better and not on negative aspects of my riding ability. Eventually, those fears and obstacles just disappeared from my mind, and I was free of unnecessary worries.

3.   Remember that we are primarily emotional animals over being rational humans. We respond to instinctive needs and then rationalize our thoughts

about them later. Praise others for their small successes and give them small but meaningful incentives to help them continue improving. Create a system where you evaluate and reward each other for accomplishments of specific tasks. Build confidence within yourself and help others build confidence in themselves.

4. Create many preventative measures in advance and avoid unnecessary conflicts. This way, you and your coworkers can focus on the task itself and work hard. With a cooperative spirit, you can work together and overcome many difficulties. Risk management is nothing but taking a number of preventative measures.

5. Have a meeting on a regular basis. Meeting regularly with another person helps you check your employees' status and give them the next achievable goal. As an added benefit, your employees will think together, help each other and watch out for each other. This way, they have more eyes watching themselves. Just letting them talk about different work strategies and goals over some tea, coffee, or a meal will help them work with each other. You can also sort out the team players who are willing to work with you or not.

6. Draw out your directions from your employees' own words instead of

always giving them direct orders. In other words, lead them to thinking about what needs to be done through a discussion. This way, you can be sure that your employees are doing the right work and they are willing to do it. Let them participate in figuring out what needs to be done. Orders are not as welcome as the person's own thoughts. Leave them some time and space to think, plan, and work on their own. Let other employees see what others are doing and how they go about it. However, you do not have to micromanage your employees. Just as you can plan your steps through the most logical thinking process, so can your employees. When, it is their idea, they will work even harder to execute it.

7.   Remember, just as you chose to be positive, others also have to choose to be positive and happy. Many people in this world have been trained by others or have trained themselves to be negative. Avoid these people and remain happy. Only keep those who are only willing to be happy with you as friends.

BONUS 2: MY READING LIST

MY READING LIST

1. Don't worry make money by Richard Carlson

2. Don't sweat the small stuff by Richard Carlson

3. Rich Dad Poor Dad by Robert Kiyosaki

4. Think and Grow Rich by Napoleon Hill

5. The Millionaire Next Door by Thomas J. Stanley Ph.D.

6. How to Win Friends and Influence People by Dale Carnegie

7. Seven Habits of Highly Successful People by Stephen R. Covey

8. The 12 Factors of Business Success by Kevin Hogan, Dave Lakhani, and Mollie Marti

9. Awaken the Giant Within by Anthony Robbins

10. The Alchemist by Paolo Coelho

11. The Little Prince by Antoine de Saint-Exupéry

12. Who Moved My cheese? by Spencer Johnson and Kenneth Blanchard

13. Chicken Soup for the Soul by Jack Canfield and Mark Victor Hansen

14. Life Without Limits by Nick Vujicic

15. One Meal a Day by Nagumo Yoshinori, MD

16. How to be a fierce competitor by Jeffrefy J. Fox

ABOUT THE AUTHOR

Ben Frank is a bestselling author in success and self-development. He has a Ph.D in education and has given many lectures in colleges and institutions. He is fluent in four languages and manages a number of successful businesses. Even though he is mainly an educator, he has strong interest in success literature. This is his second book in his success and self-development series, "The Life Success." His previous best seller is "Positive Thinking Power: How to live a stress free life with confidence, happiness, and Joy (Five Simple Steps to a positive lifestyle). He is living happily with his wife and two children. To find more about him, you can visit www.thelifesuccess.com (coming soon).

www.ingramcontent.com/pod-product-compliance
Lightning Source LLC
Chambersburg PA
CBHW071130280526
45787CB00003B/1235